Misty Wesley

What any women should know about Breast Cancer

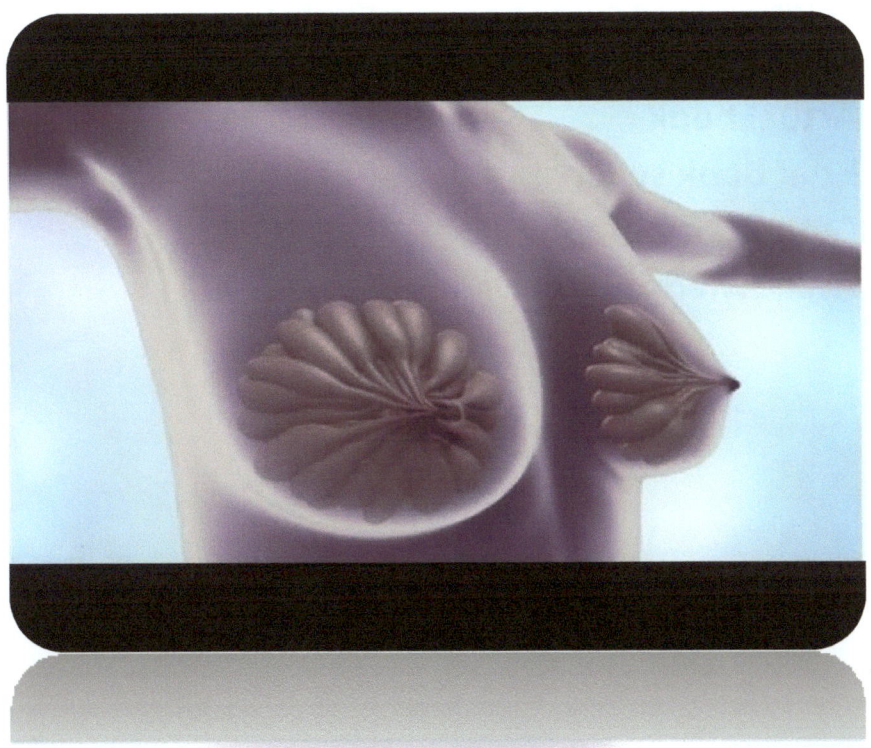

1

Table of Contents

Dedication's Page

This book is dedicated to all of my family members, friends, and patients who has been diagnosed with this deadly disease.

Always remember that you are a fighter!!!

A cancer that develops from breast tissue is defined as Breast Cancer.
Some significant signs of Breast Cancer may be a change in breast shape, a lump in the breast, nipple dimpling (nipple moves inward), nipple secretions, or a red scaly patch of skin around the breast.

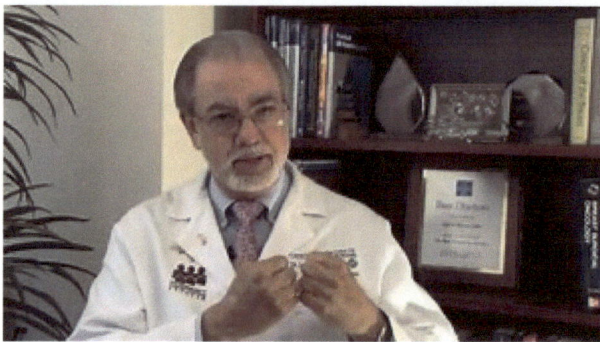

With those individuals who have a history of already having Breast Cancer, they can also have yellow skin, shortness of air, and skeletal pain.

The first sign of an individual having breast cancer may be an abnormal mammogram or a lump in their breast. Men do not often get Breast Cancer and it is uncommon but not unheard of yet it still must be taken seriously.

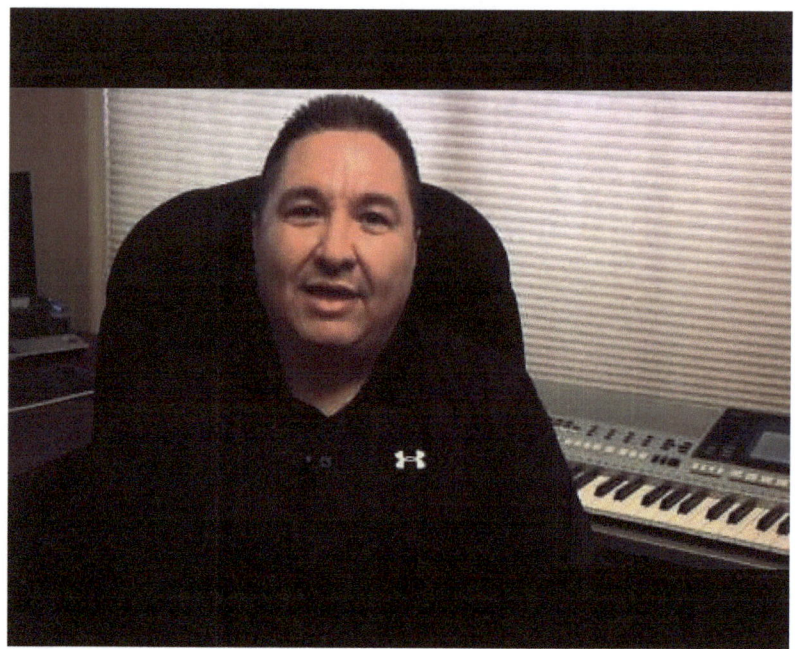

Misty Wesley

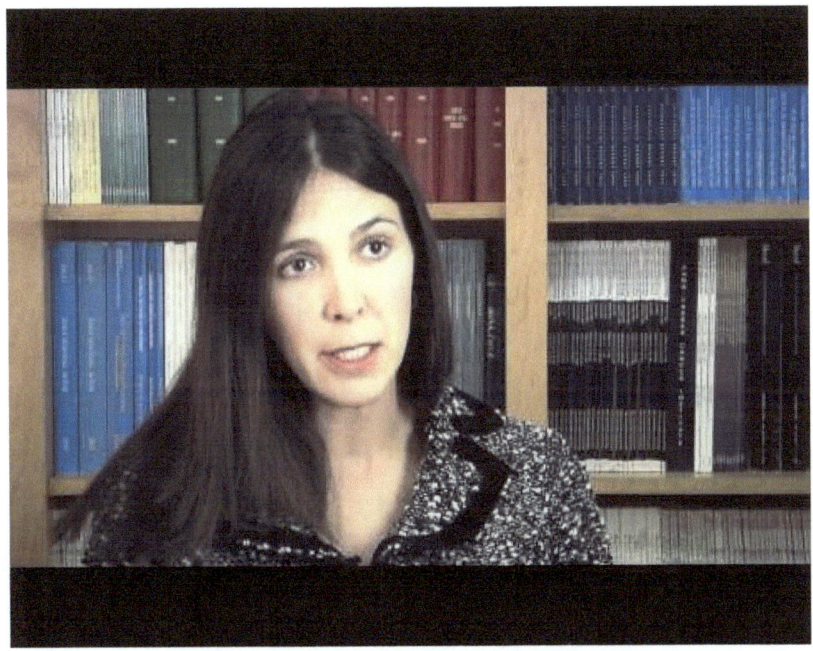

Some of the stages of Breast Cancer

Some of the stages of Breast Cancer may be:

➢ **Early**
➢ **Curable Breast Cancer**
➢ **Metastatic Breast Cancer with a variety of treatments available**

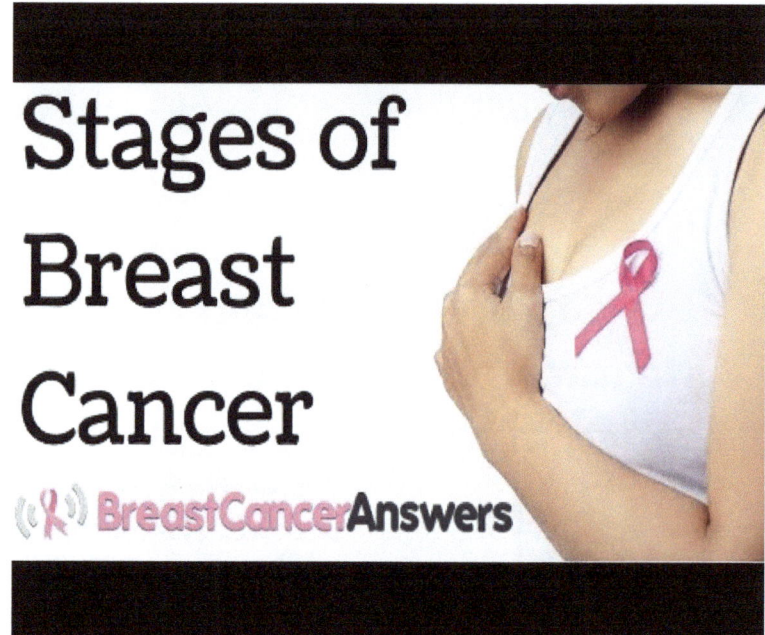

Breast Cancer Symptoms and Types

Generally, most breast lumps are not cancerous.

A breast lump isn't the only warning sign for Breast Cancer.

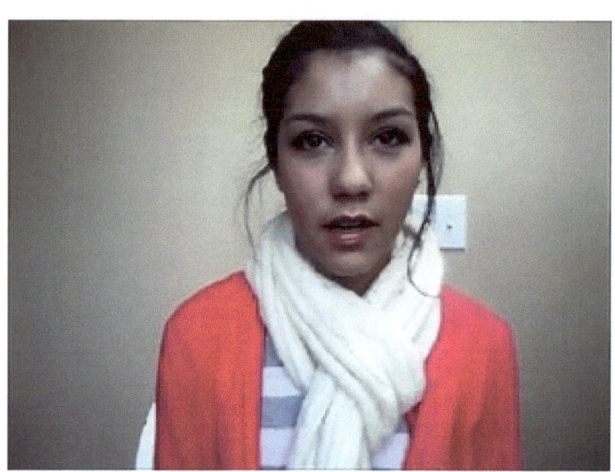

Breast Cancer Symptoms

Breast Cancer patients generally have no symptoms while the cancer is in its early stages. When a patient has a tumor develop, they generally may have these types of symptoms:

❖ A lump in the breast or underneath the arm

❖ Edema or swelling in the axilla or armpit region

❖ Breast pain and tenderness

❖ A noticeable indentation or flattening on the breast area

❖ A temperature, texture, contour, or size of the breast

❖ Nipple changes of any type

❖ Unusual discharge from the nipple of any type or color

❖ A marble-like area underneath the skin's surface

❖ An area of the breast that is distinctly different than any other area or region

Consulting your physician after you have been diagnosed with Breast Cancer

A person should always consult their physician when:
1) Swollen lymph glands in the armpit regions
2) When one or both breasts develop persistent pain, develop lumps or the breasts look or even feel abnormal

Breast Cancer Detection and Treatments

**Breast Cancer is best diagnosed by early detection.
A patient's long-term health can be greatly extended by the early detection of Breast Cancer.
So please get your mammogram!!!**

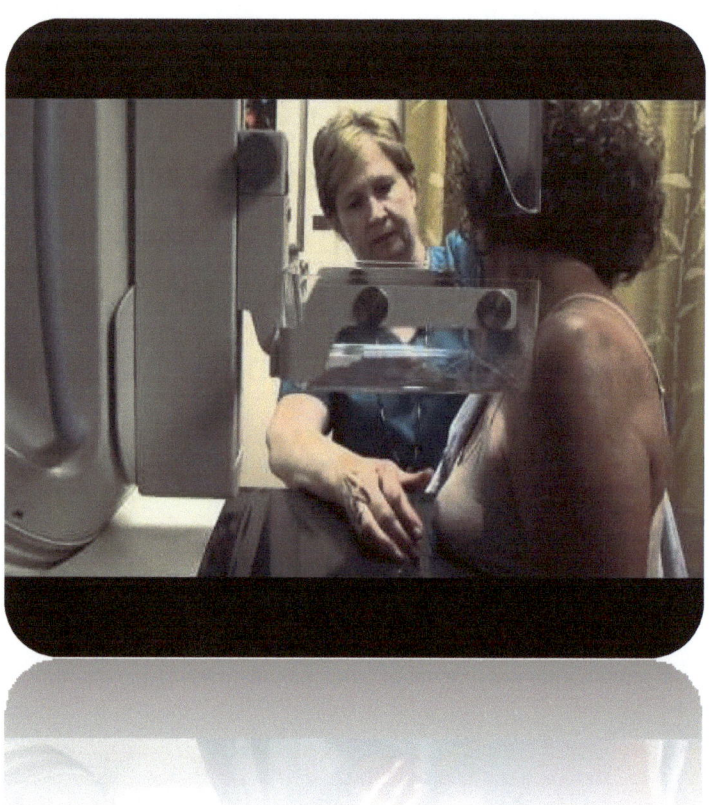

Breast Cancer Screening:

What kind and when???

Misty Wesley

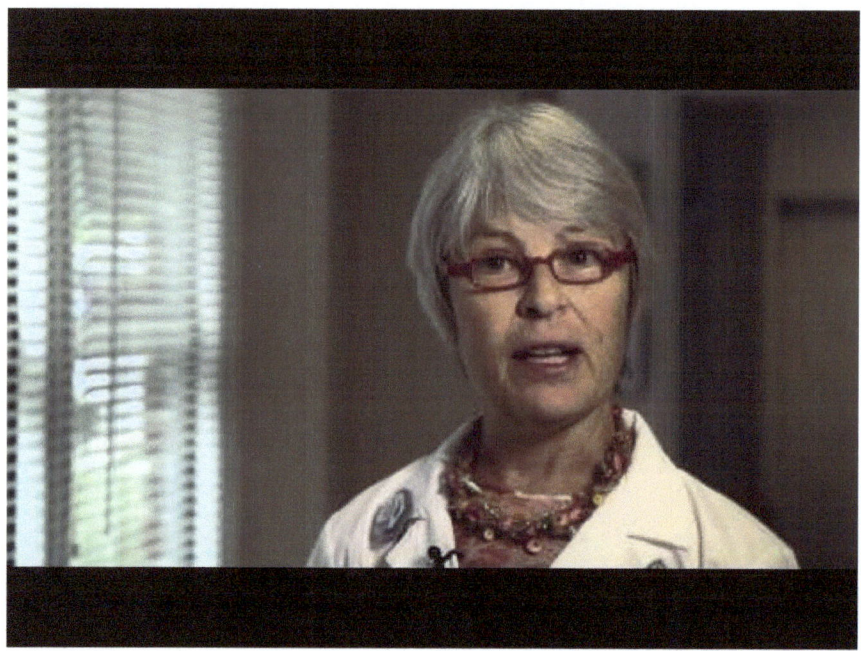

For women or men that fall into the normal risk range, they can perform self-examinations, have a mammogram performed, and have clinical examinations starting at the age of 40.

For women or men that fall into the high-risk range, they may have to have additional tests such as an MRI of the Breast, an ultrasound of the Breast or a nuclear test done.

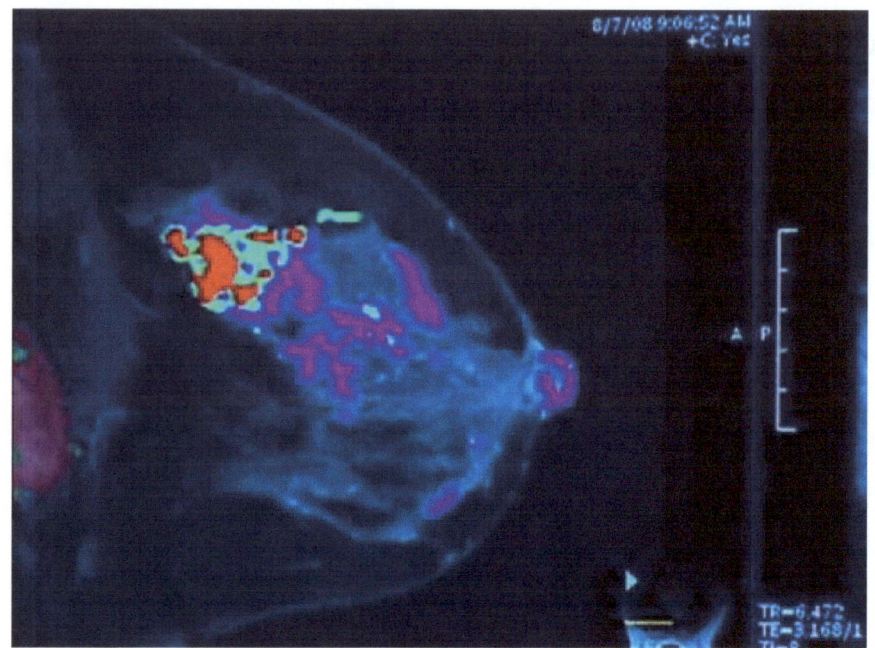

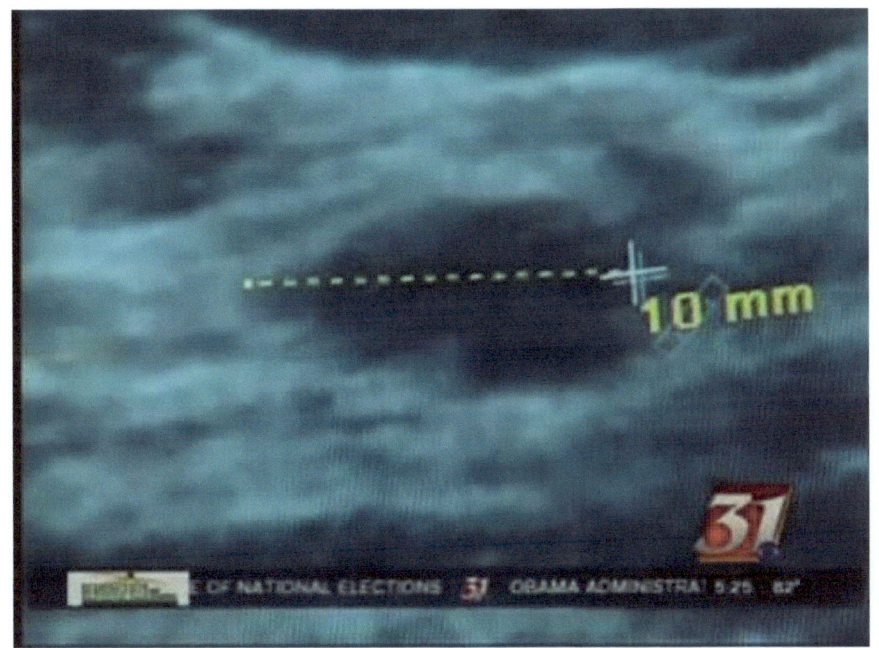

Misty Wesley

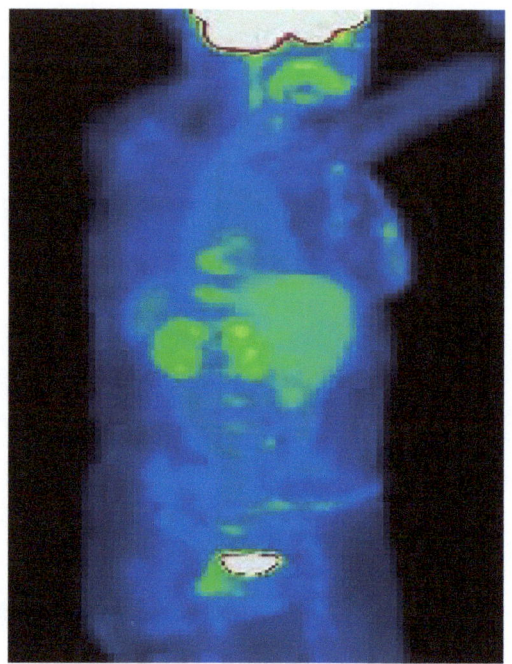

Breast Cancer Procedures that may be conducted

Some patients have no unearthly idea as to what will happen when a mammogram is scheduled such as:

- **Always perform self-examinations on yourself**
- **A physician could schedule a mammogram for you**
- **Your physician will always perform a clinical examination starting at the age of 20**
- **A breast biopsy may be performed**
- **An ultrasound of the breast**
- **A MRI of the breast**
- **Sentinel node biopsy of the breast**
- **Ductal lavage of the breast to check for precancerous cells of any kind**

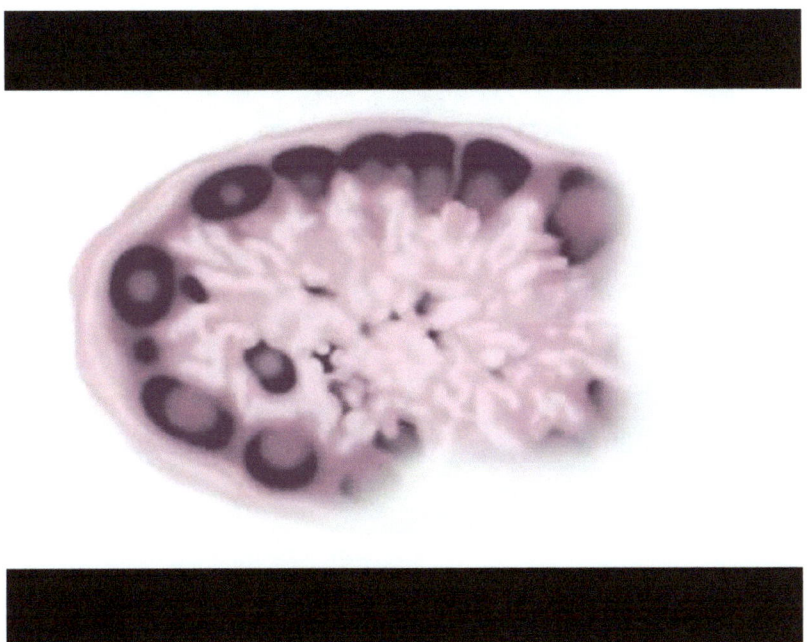

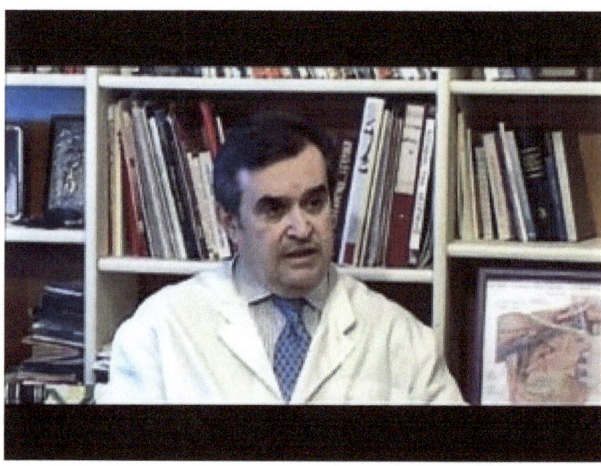

Breast Cancer Care and Some Treatments that may be available in your area

Did you know that there are over 2 million Breast Cancer survivors in the United States today? Modern medicine and its updated techniques are some of the reasons for this great success and the main reason are the Breast Cancer survivors themselves who fight for the right to live!

Breast Cancer treatments have come a long way over the years, so here are some of the most common treatments that could be available:

- ✓ Find the right healthcare facility and physician that you actually like
  - ✓ Breast Cancer surgery
  - ✓ Chemotherapy
  - ✓ Radiation of the Breast
  - ✓ Hormone therapy
  - ✓ Hormone drug therapy
- ✓ Biological therapy for Breast Cancer
  - ✓ Herceptin
- ✓ Treating your Breast Cancer by its stage of development
  - ✓ Follow-up care for your Breast Cancer
  - ✓ Recurrent Breast Cancer Treatments
- ✓ Alternative Medicines and Complimentary Therapies for Breast Cancer

Breast Cancer Care

Misty Wesley

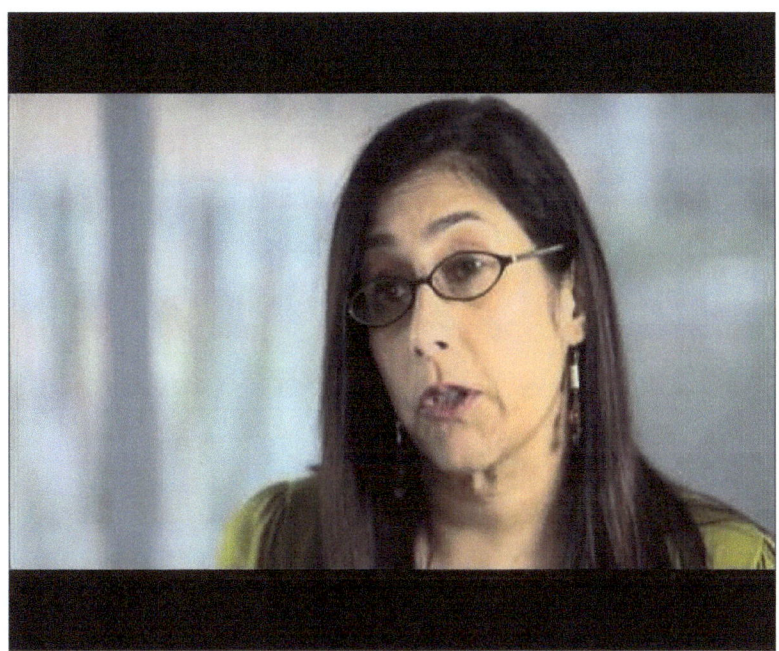

There are several types of follow-up care for Breast Cancer Survivors and here are just a couple of examples:

- o **Get a second opinion**
- o **Become a proactive Breast Cancer patient**
- o **Find the best Breast Cancer physicians**
- o **Choose the best facility for you**
- o **Perform your exercises after your surgery**
- o **Debate about a new Breast Cancer clinical trial that is in your area**
- o **Try to have some fun, go to a Breast Cancer Fashion Show, remember sometimes fun and laughter could be the best medicine on a particular day**

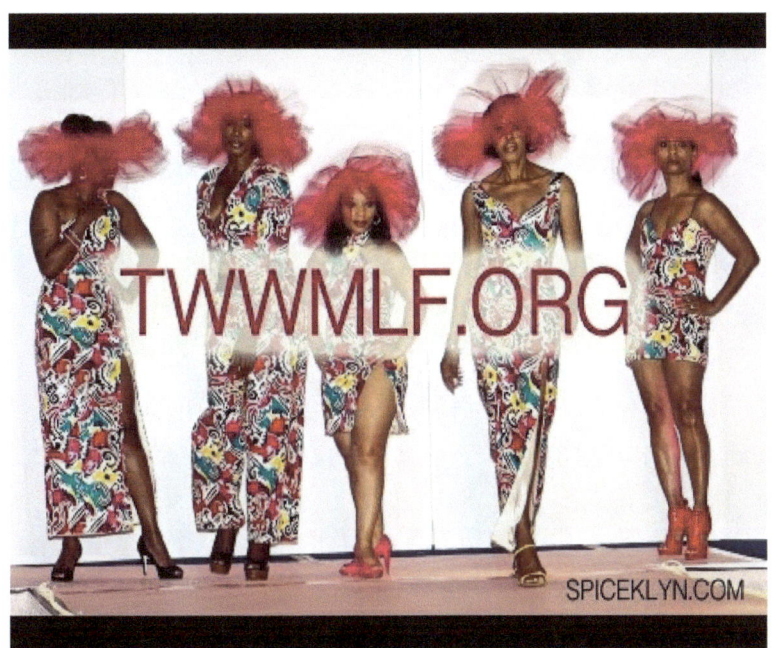

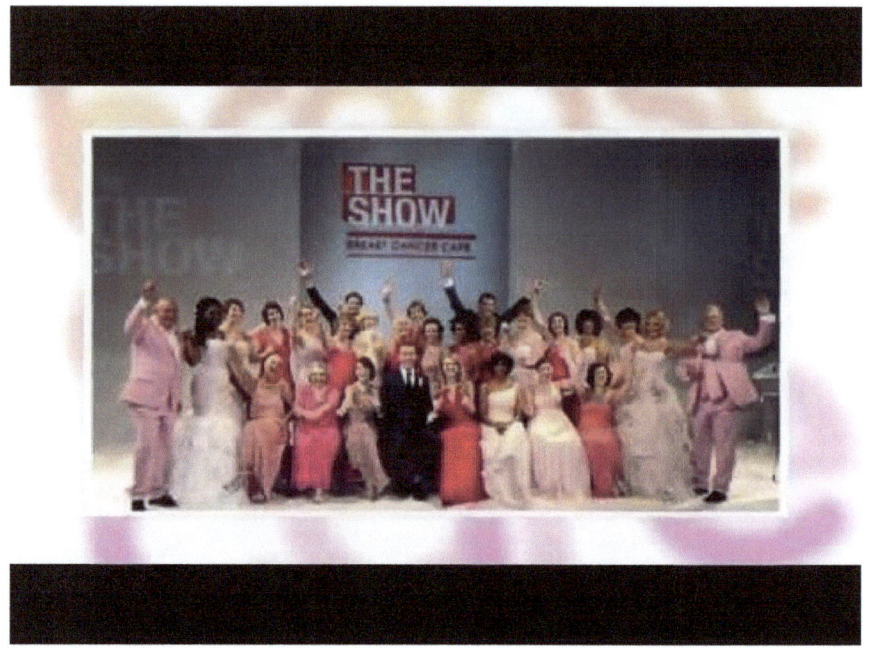

You can live and cope with your Breast Cancer Disease

A person can live, manage and cope with Breast Cancer disease.

You may have to learn to manage the cancer fatigue. How a person does this is basically up to the individual and their hectic schedules.

An individual can also look into Breast Reconstructive Surgery and they can learn how to manage their diet and exercise routines.

The patients could also join a Breast Cancer friendship board to.

Remember, your possibilities are endless once you set your mind to a speedy recovery!

Conclusions

The author openly admits that she could never imagine what Breast Cancer patients go through but she wants all of her family, friends and patients to know that she admires all of them more than they could ever possibly imagine.

To look death in the face and then smile while trying to defeat it well, words just can't describe the ordeal.

The author wants everyone to know that her family members, friends and all of her patients were her true inspirations in writing this book.

She hopes that you find the book helpful and informative!

The End

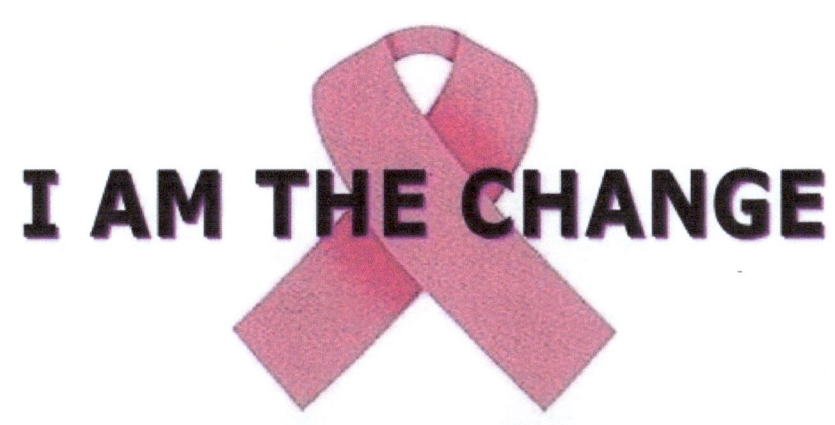

This Breast Cancer book is an informative self-help manual that gives people an overview of Breast Cancer, some of its treatments and procedures that may be ordered or performed, describes some treatments that may be used and gives you some healthcare tips on how to manage and actually cope with the Breast Cancer disease. The author has also included some very informative and professional videos which will only be on the digital formatted version of the book that she hopes will further explain the Breast Cancer disease. The beginning of the videos will only be included in the book format. God bless!

Misty Lynn Wesley has a diversified career portfolio in the medical, legal, fashion and insurance industries. She is an avid blogger for Examiner.com, Helium, and Yahoo Voices. She is a published author for Publish America and Create Space. She has been in the medical field

For over 20 years and her family members, friends and patients were her true inspirations in writing this book. She truly hopes that you will enjoy the book with the neat videos that are embedded in this digital book. God bless!

Acknowledgements

This digital are and embedded videos are courtesy of the following:

1) www.publicdomaindigitalart.net
2) www.youtube.com/rontho
3) www.youtube.com/mayoclinic
4) www.youtube.com/mountainevent12
5) www.youtube.com/Idiscoveredalumpinmybreast
6) www.youtube.com/dryayharness
7) www.youtube.com/QVCBreastCancerAwareness
8) www.youtube.com/spicekyln
9) www.youtube.com/iamthechange

Let this legal record reflect that there are no contracts on You Tube to visualize before uploading the videos. The author has given credit to the contractor. Any person, entity, or corporation should evaluate the Good Samaritan Law before any Arbitration or Civil Suit is pursued!